MASTERING MEDICAL TERMINILOGY

Your KEY TO UNDERSTANDING HEALTHCARE LANGUAGE

ALEX USIFO

To all those who tirelessly dedicate their lives to the well-being of others, this book is a humble tribute to your unwavering compassion and dedication.

To the patients, whose resilience and trust inspire us to continually strive for medical excellence and better healthcare outcomes. Your strength is our motivation.

To my mentors and colleagues, who have shared their knowledge and experiences, shaping my journey in the world of medicine. Your guidance has been invaluable.

To my family, for their endless support, understanding, and patience during the long hours of research and writing. Your love sustains me.

And finally, to the countless individuals who will read these pages in search of understanding, answers, or hope. May this book serve as a source of knowledge and empowerment in your medical journey.

With deep appreciation and a profound sense of purpose,

CONTENTS

Introduction

In the vast and intricate world of medicine, where the language can often seem like an enigma to the uninitiated, one fundamental key unlocks the door to understanding and communication: medical terminology. This book, "Medical Terminology: A Comprehensive Guide," is your essential companion on a journey through the intricacies of this language, unraveling its codes, and empowering you to navigate the realm of healthcare with confidence and precision.

Medical terminology is the language of healthcare professionals. It serves as a universal means of communication, enabling physicians, nurses, pharmacists, and all those involved in the healthcare field to convey complex concepts, procedures, and conditions succinctly and accurately. Beyond professionals, a grasp of medical terminology equips patients with the knowledge they need to engage in informed discussions about their health.

Our journey begins by delving into the very foundations of medical terminology. We will explore the structure of medical words, examining roots, prefixes, and suffixes, to decode the meaning of complex terms. From there, we'll venture into the vast landscape of anatomical terminology, dissecting the human body into its constituent parts, positions, and planes.

In Chapter 2, we'll decipher the multitude of abbreviations and symbols used in medical documentation. You'll gain the ability to interpret medical charts, prescriptions, and clinical notes with ease.

Diagnostic procedures and medical specialties take center stage in

Chapter 3. We'll unravel the language of medical tests, imaging, and the diverse medical specialties, from cardiology to radiology.

Disease and conditions, the crux of medical terminology, become our focus in Chapter 4. You'll learn how to name diseases, conditions, and their various manifestations, utilizing prefixes and suffixes as your linguistic tools.

Pharmacy and medication are essential components of healthcare, and Chapter 5 introduces you to the terminology associated with drug names, classifications, and prescription writing.

Surgical procedures, medical equipment and technology, and the intricate language of body systems are all dissected in their respective chapters. You'll become proficient in understanding the tools of the trade and the lexicon that accompanies them.

In Chapter 10, we explore the unique prefixes and suffixes specific to each body system, providing you with a comprehensive understanding of how medical terms are crafted.

The book is not only a theoretical exploration but a practical guide. Chapter 9 presents practice exercises to reinforce your learning, enabling you to confidently wield your newfound knowledge.

Chapter 12 places you in real-world scenarios, showcasing the practical applications of medical terminology and its role in patient care.

Ethical and cultural considerations in medical terminology are addressed in Chapter `11 and 12 emphasizing the importance of clear, respectful, and sensitive communication in the healthcare field.

As we look ahead in Chapter 12, we consider the future trends in medical terminology, recognizing the impact of advances in medicine and technology on this evolving language.

With "Medical Terminology: A Comprehensive Guide," you're equipped to decode the language of healthcare, improving your ability to communicate, learn, and engage in the fascinating world of medicine. Together, we'll embark on a journey of discovery, one word at a time, and empower you to be a knowledgeable and confident participant in the field of healthcare.

CHAPTER 1

Basic Word Structure

Medical terminology is a structured language with a precise construction that allows for clear and accurate communication. In this chapter, we'll explore the foundational elements of medical terminology, including word roots, prefixes, and suffixes. These components are the building blocks of medical words and serve as the key to unlocking the meanings of complex terms.

Section 1: Word Roots

Definition: The word root is the foundation of a medical term.

It typically comes from Latin or Greek and conveys the primary meaning of the word.

Examples: Common word roots include "cardio," meaning heart, and "derm," meaning skin.

Word Root Modification: Sometimes, word roots can be modified by changing their form or combining them with other word roots to create more specific terms.

Section 2: Prefixes

Definition: A prefix is a word part added to the beginning of a word to modify its meaning. In medical terminology, prefixes provide additional context to the word.

Examples: "Hypo-" means below or deficient, so "hypotension" refers to low blood pressure.

Prefixes for Quantity and Measurement: Some prefixes denote quantity or measurement, like "micro-" (small) or "macro-" (large).

Section 3: Suffixes

Definition: A suffix is a word part added to the end of a word to modify its meaning. In medical terminology, suffixes often indicate a procedure, condition, or disease.

Examples: "Itis" is a common suffix meaning inflammation, as in "tonsillitis" (inflammation of the tonsils).

Suffixes for Procedures: Suffixes like "-ectomy" (removal) and "-plasty" (surgical repair) are used to describe medical procedures.

Section 4: Building Medical Terms

Combining Word Parts: Medical terms are constructed by combining word roots, prefixes, and suffixes. For example, "cardiologist" combines "cardio" (heart) and "logist" (one who studies), meaning a specialist who studies the heart.

Understanding Terminology: Breaking down medical terms into

their components makes it easier to understand their meanings and memorize a vast array of terms.

Pronunciation and Spelling Rules: Learning how to pronounce medical terms correctly and following specific spelling rules are essential for precise communication.

CHAPTER 2

Anatomical Terminology

Anatomy is the study of the structure of the human body, and medical professionals rely on a specialized language to accurately describe its components, positions, and movements. In this chapter, we will explore the key anatomical terminology that forms the basis for understanding the human body's structure and organization.

Section 1: Body Planes and Positions

Anatomical Position: The standardized reference position used in anatomy, where the body is standing upright, arms at the sides, and palms facing forward.

Body Planes: Anatomical planes are imaginary lines used to divide the body for reference. Common planes include the sagittal plane, frontal (coronal) plane, and transverse (horizontal) plane.

Body Directions: Terms like "anterior" (front), "posterior" (back), "superior" (above), and "inferior" (below) are used to describe the relative positions of body parts.

Section 2: Regional Anatomy

Body Regions: The body is divided into regions for specific reference. These include the head, neck, trunk, and extremities.

Quadrants and Regions: The abdomen, for example, is divided into four quadrants and nine regions to precisely describe the location of organs and structures.

Section 3: Anatomical Structures

Body Systems: The human body is organized into various systems, such as the circulatory system, respiratory system, and nervous system. Understanding these systems is crucial for describing anatomical structures and functions.

Major Organs and Structures: In this section, you will learn the names and locations of major organs and structures in the body, including the heart, lungs, brain, and more.

Section 4: Anatomical Directions and Movements

Flexion and Extension: Flexion refers to bending a joint, while extension is the straightening of a joint.

Abduction and Adduction: Abduction involves moving a body part away from the midline, while adduction brings it back toward the midline.

Rotation and Circumduction: Rotation is the turning of a bone around its own axis, while circumduction is a circular movement of a limb.

Section 5: Specialized Terminology

Terms for Bones and Joints: Understanding terms like "femur" (thigh bone) and "humerus" (upper arm bone) is vital for discussing the skeletal system.

Muscular Terminology: Learning the names of muscles and their actions, such as "biceps" and "quadriceps," is essential for discussions related to the muscular system.

Vascular and Nervous System Terms: Familiarity with terms like "artery," "vein," "neuron," and "cerebellum" is important when discussing the vascular and nervous systems.

Section 6: Clinical and Diagnostic Terminology

Radiological Terms: Understanding terms used in medical imaging, like "MRI" (Magnetic Resonance Imaging) and "CT scan" (Computed Tomography scan).

Medical Procedures: Knowledge of terms used during medical procedures, such as "arthroscopy" (a minimally invasive procedure to examine the inside of a joint).

CHAPTER 3

Medical Abbreviations and Symbols

In the fast-paced world of healthcare, abbreviations and symbols play a crucial role in simplifying documentation, communication, and record-keeping. However, their extensive use also requires healthcare professionals to be well-versed in their meanings to ensure accurate and safe patient care. In this chapter, we will explore common medical abbreviations and symbols and the contexts in which they are employed.

Section 1: The Importance of Medical Abbreviations

Efficient Communication: Medical abbreviations save time and space in documentation, which is especially vital in emergency situations or when recording patient information.

Reducing Errors: While abbreviations are efficient, their misuse can lead to errors. Understanding them and adhering to standard practices is essential for patient safety.

Section 2: Common Medical Abbreviations

Rx: Abbreviation for "prescription." It indicates that a medication is to be dispensed.

PRN: Short for "pro re nata," meaning "as needed." This abbreviation is often used in medication orders.

NPO: Abbreviation for "nil per os," indicating that a patient should not consume any food or liquids orally.

ADL: Stands for "activities of daily living," describing a person's ability to perform routine self-care tasks.

STAT: An abbreviation that indicates something should be done immediately.

BMI: Acronym for "body mass index," a measure of body fat based on height and weight.

Section 3: Medical Symbols

Medical Alert Symbol: The medical alert symbol, often a red caduceus, is used to indicate a medical condition or allergy.

Prescription Symbol: The symbol "℞" is widely recognized as a prescription symbol, indicating a medication order.

Medical Degrees and Units: Understanding symbols like °F (degrees Fahrenheit) or mg (milligrams) is crucial for accurate dosage and patient care.

Section 4: Acronyms and Initialisms

HMO: Stands for "health maintenance organization," a type of managed care plan.

ICU: Abbreviation for "intensive care unit," a specialized department in hospitals.

CPR: Acronym for "cardiopulmonary resuscitation," an emergency life-saving procedure.

AIDS: Acronym for "acquired immunodeficiency syndrome," a condition caused by HIV.

Section 5: Medical Records and Documentation

Electronic Health Records (EHRs): Electronic medical records have introduced a new set of abbreviations and symbols, impacting the way patient information is recorded and accessed.

Standard Abbreviations: There are many standard abbreviations and symbols used in medical documentation to maintain consistency and clarity.

Section 6: Challenges and Solutions

Abbreviation Errors: The potential for misinterpretation and errors associated with abbreviations and symbols in healthcare.

Solutions and Best Practices: Recommendations for healthcare professionals to reduce the risks of abbreviation-related errors.

CHAPTER 4

Diagnostic Procedures and Medical Specialties

In the dynamic world of healthcare, diagnostic procedures and specialized medical fields play a crucial role in understanding and treating a wide range of conditions. In this chapter, we will explore the diverse diagnostic procedures used to identify diseases and conditions and introduce some of the key medical specialties and their associated terminology.

Section 1: Diagnostic Procedures

Physical Examination: A fundamental diagnostic tool that involves the systematic assessment of a patient's body to identify signs of disease or dysfunction.

Laboratory Tests: Diagnostic tests that analyze various bodily fluids and tissues, including blood tests, urine analysis, and biopsies.

Medical Imaging: Techniques such as X-rays, CT scans, MRI, and ultrasound that create visual representations of the inside of the body.

Endoscopy: A procedure that involves inserting a flexible tube with a camera into the body to examine internal organs.

Biopsy: The removal of a small tissue sample for examination, often to diagnose or rule out cancer.

Section 2: Medical Specialties

Cardiology: The branch of medicine focused on the cardiovascular system, including the heart and blood vessels.

Oncology: The field dedicated to the study and treatment of

cancer, involving various subspecialties.

Neurology: The medical specialty concerned with disorders of the nervous system, including the brain, spinal cord, and peripheral nerves.

Orthopedics: Specializing in the musculoskeletal system, including bones, joints, muscles, and tendons.

Gastroenterology: Focusing on the digestive system and gastrointestinal disorders.

Obstetrics and Gynecology (OB/GYN): A medical specialty addressing women's health, pregnancy, and childbirth.

Pediatrics: The branch of medicine that deals with the care of children, from infancy through adolescence.

Section 3: Navigating Medical Specialties

Interdisciplinary Collaboration: How different medical specialties often work together to provide comprehensive patient care.

Referrals and Consultations: The process of referring patients to specialists when a condition falls outside the expertise of the primary care provider.

Subspecialties: Within many medical specialties, there are subspecialties that focus on specific areas. For instance, in cardiology, there are subspecialties like interventional cardiology or electrophysiology.

Section 4: Terminology in Practice

Diagnostic Terminology: Understanding the terms and language used in various diagnostic procedures, such as "echocardiogram" in cardiology.

Specialty-Specific Terminology: Exploring the specialized vocabulary of different medical fields, such as "oncologist" in oncology.

Patient Education: The importance of effective communication with patients, including explaining diagnostic procedures and conditions in understandable terms.

CHAPTER 5

Diseases and Conditions

In the realm of healthcare, understanding and correctly identifying diseases and medical conditions is a fundamental aspect of medical practice. This chapter delves into the terminology associated with a wide range of diseases and conditions, enabling healthcare professionals to accurately diagnose and manage patients' health.

Section 1: Disease Naming and Classification

Nomenclature: The principles of naming diseases, often following a standardized classification system, which aids in clear communication among healthcare professionals.

International Classification of Diseases (ICD): An internationally recognized system used for coding and classifying diseases and health-related problems for statistical and billing purposes.

Section 2: Common Diseases and Conditions

Cardiovascular Conditions: Understanding diseases like hypertension, myocardial infarction, and congestive heart failure, which affect the heart and blood vessels.

Respiratory Diseases: Knowledge of conditions such as asthma, chronic obstructive pulmonary disease (COPD), and pneumonia, which impact the respiratory system.

Infectious Diseases: Terminology for diseases caused by infectious agents, including viruses, bacteria, and fungi, such as tuberculosis, HIV/AIDS, and influenza.

Autoimmune Disorders: Conditions where the immune system attacks the body's own tissues, like rheumatoid arthritis and multiple sclerosis.

Endocrine Disorders: Understanding diseases affecting the endocrine system, such as diabetes, hyperthyroidism, and hypothyroidism.

Section 3: Specialized Conditions and Terminology

Cancer Terminology: The nomenclature and classification of different types of cancer, such as carcinoma, sarcoma, and lymphoma.

Psychiatric Disorders: Understanding terms related to mental health conditions, including depression, anxiety disorders, and schizophrenia.

Genetic Disorders: Terminology associated with genetic conditions like Down syndrome, cystic fibrosis, and Huntington's disease.

Section 4: Infectious Diseases and Outbreaks

Epidemics and Pandemics: Definitions and distinctions between epidemics (outbreaks of a disease in a specific region) and pandemics (global outbreaks).

Contagious Diseases: Understanding the characteristics and terminology of highly contagious diseases, like measles and COVID-19.

Vaccination: Key terminology related to vaccines and immunization, essential in the prevention and control of infectious diseases.

Section 5: Chronic Conditions and Lifestyle-Related Diseases

Lifestyle Diseases: A look at diseases often associated with lifestyle choices, such as heart disease, obesity, and type 2 diabetes.

Chronic Conditions: Terminology related to long-term, often incurable diseases, such as chronic obstructive pulmonary disease (COPD) and kidney disease.

Section 6: Patient Education and Communication

Explaining Diagnoses: The importance of healthcare professionals effectively communicating with patients to explain their diagnoses, using understandable language.

Support and Coping: The role of medical professionals in providing support and coping strategies for patients diagnosed with serious or chronic conditions.

Oral Medications: Terms related to drugs taken by mouth, including "per os" (by mouth) and "sublingual" (under the tongue).

Injections: The vocabulary associated with various injection types, such as "intramuscular" and "intravenous."

Topical Medications: Terminology for drugs applied to the skin or mucous membranes, including "transdermal" and "intranasal."

Section 4: Medication Interactions and Side Effects

Drug-Drug Interactions: Terminology for interactions between different medications that can affect their effectiveness or safety.

Adverse Effects: Terms describing side effects, adverse reactions, and contraindications associated with medications.

Section 5: Pharmacy Practice and Terminology

Pharmacists and Pharmacy Technicians: The roles of healthcare professionals in the field of pharmacy, including their education and responsibilities.

Dispensing and Compounding: Terms related to the preparation and distribution of medications in the pharmacy setting.

Pharmacy Regulations and Laws: An overview of the laws and

regulations that govern the practice of pharmacy, including the Controlled Substances Act.

Section 6: Patient Education and Medication Management

Medication Adherence: The importance of patients following prescribed medication regimens, and the role of healthcare providers in educating patients.

Medication Safety: Strategies to ensure the safe and responsible use of medications, including proper storage and disposal.

CHAPTER 6

Surgical Procedures

Surgical procedures are a vital component of healthcare, offering both diagnostic and therapeutic solutions for various medical conditions. This chapter explores the terminology and procedures related to surgery, providing healthcare professionals with the essential language to understand, communicate, and participate in the surgical aspects of patient care.

Section 1: Surgical Specialties

General Surgery: A broad surgical specialty covering a wide range of procedures, including appendectomies, hernia repairs, and cholecystectomies.

Orthopedic Surgery: Focused on the musculoskeletal system, including procedures like joint replacements and fracture repairs.

Cardiothoracic Surgery: Specializing in surgeries of the heart and chest, such as coronary artery bypass grafting (CABG) and lung resections.

Neurosurgery: Concentrating on surgical interventions of the nervous system, including brain and spinal surgeries.

Gynecological Surgery: Surgical procedures related to the female reproductive system, like hysterectomies and ovarian cyst removal.

Section 2: Surgical Procedures and Techniques

Incisions and Approaches: Terminology associated with surgical incisions, such as "midline incision" or "laparoscopic approach."

Surgical Instruments: The names and uses of instruments like scalpels, forceps, and retractors.

Anesthesia: Understanding the types of anesthesia used in surgery, including general anesthesia, regional anesthesia, and local anesthesia.

Suture Types: Vocabulary related to different suture materials and techniques, like "interrupted sutures" and "continuous sutures."

Section 3: Preoperative and Postoperative Care

Preoperative Evaluation: The assessment of a patient's condition before surgery, involving terms like "NPO" (nothing by mouth) and "consent forms."

Postoperative Recovery: Understanding postoperative care, including terms like "post-anesthesia care unit (PACU)" and "discharge instructions."

Complications and Adverse Events: Terminology related to potential surgical complications, such as "infection" and "thrombosis."

Section 4: Emerging Surgical Technologies

Minimally Invasive Surgery: Terminology associated with minimally invasive techniques, like laparoscopy and robotic surgery.

Telemedicine in Surgery: The impact of telemedicine on surgical consultations, preoperative evaluations, and postoperative follow-up.

Section 5: Patient Communication and Informed Consent

Informed Consent: Explaining the concept of informed consent to patients and ensuring they understand the risks and benefits of surgical procedures.

Patient Education: The importance of patient education before surgery, including discussing the procedure and what to expect during the surgical journey.

CHAPTER 7

Medical Equipment and Technology

Medical technology and equipment are at the forefront of healthcare, enabling accurate diagnoses and effective treatments. This chapter delves into the terminology associated with medical equipment and technology, providing healthcare professionals with the language to understand, operate, and communicate about these vital tools.

Section 1: Diagnostic and Imaging Equipment

X-ray Machines: Understanding the terminology related to radiography and the use of X-rays for imaging.

Magnetic Resonance Imaging (MRI): The vocabulary associated with MRI technology, which uses powerful magnets and radio waves to create detailed images of the body.

Computed Tomography (CT) Scanners: Terminology specific to CT scans, which use X-rays and computer technology to produce cross-sectional images of the body.

Ultrasound Equipment: Terminology for ultrasound devices that use high-frequency sound waves to visualize structures within the body.

Section 2: Laboratory and Diagnostic Tools

Microscopes: Vocabulary related to microscopes used in pathology and laboratory settings to examine tissues and microorganisms.

Stethoscopes: Understanding the components and use of stethoscopes in clinical assessments.

Electrocardiography (ECG or EKG): The terminology associated with ECG equipment for monitoring and recording electrical activity of the heart.

Pulse Oximeters: Vocabulary related to pulse oximeters, devices used to measure oxygen saturation in the blood.

Section 3: Life Support and Monitoring Equipment

Ventilators: Terminology for ventilators, machines that assist with breathing by delivering air and oxygen to the lungs.

Cardiac Monitors: Understanding the terminology of cardiac monitoring equipment used to track heart rate and rhythm.

Defibrillators: Vocabulary related to defibrillators, devices that deliver an electric shock to restore normal heart rhythm.

Section 4: Surgical and Medical Instruments

Scalpels and Surgical Instruments: Understanding the names and uses of surgical instruments like scalpels, forceps, and scissors.

Endoscopes: Terminology associated with endoscopes, instruments used to visualize and operate within the body's cavities.

Infusion Pumps: Vocabulary related to infusion pumps used to deliver fluids, medications, and nutrients to patients.

Section 5: Electronic Health Records (EHRs) and Health Information Technology

EHR Terminology: Understanding key terms in electronic health records, such as "Health Information Exchange (HIE)" and "Interoperability."

Telemedicine Technology: Vocabulary related to telemedicine technology, which enables remote patient care and consultations.

Section 6: Emerging Medical Technologies

Artificial Intelligence (AI) in Healthcare: The impact of AI and machine learning on healthcare, including terminology related to

AI applications.

Medical Robotics: Terminology associated with medical robots used in surgery, diagnostics, and patient care.

Respiratory Anatomy: Terminology for the parts of the respiratory system, including the lungs, bronchi, and alveoli.

Breathing and Gas Exchange: Understanding the processes of inhalation, exhalation, and gas exchange in the lungs.

Section 5: The Digestive System

Digestive Anatomy: Vocabulary related to the structures of the digestive system, such as the esophagus, stomach, and intestines.

Nutrient Processing: Terms for the breakdown and absorption of nutrients, including digestion and absorption.

Section 6: The Nervous System

Nervous System Anatomy: Understanding the components of the nervous system, including the brain, spinal cord, and peripheral nerves.

Neurological Processes: Vocabulary related to neurological functions, such as neurotransmission and reflexes.

Section 7: The Endocrine System

Endocrine Glands: Terminology for endocrine glands like the pituitary gland, thyroid, and adrenal glands.

Hormones and Regulation: Understanding hormone names and their roles in regulating bodily functions.

Section 8: The Reproductive System

Male and Female Reproductive Anatomy: Vocabulary related to the structures of the male and female reproductive systems, including the testes, ovaries, and uterus.

Reproductive Processes: Terms associated with reproduction, including fertilization, pregnancy, and childbirth.

Section 9: The Urinary System

Urinary Anatomy: Understanding the structures of the urinary system, including the kidneys, ureters, bladder, and urethra.

Urine Formation and Excretion: Vocabulary related to the processes of urine formation and excretion.

Section 10: The Lymphatic and Immune Systems

Lymphatic System: Terminology for lymphatic organs, vessels, and nodes, including the tonsils and spleen.

Immune Function: Vocabulary related to immune system components, like white blood cells and antibodies.

CHAPTER 8

Prefixes and Suffixes for Body Systems

Medical terminology often includes prefixes and suffixes that are added to root words to modify their meanings, particularly when describing the body's various systems. This chapter will delve into the common prefixes and suffixes used in medical terms related to body systems, providing healthcare professionals with a deeper understanding of this language.

Section 1: Common Prefixes for Body Systems

Cardio-: Pertaining to the heart. Example: Cardiovascular.

Hemo- or Hema-: Relating to blood. Example: Hematology.

Neuro-: Associated with the nervous system. Example: Neurology.

Gastro-: Involving the stomach or the gastrointestinal system. Example: Gastroenterology.

Pulmo- or Pulmono-: Relating to the lungs. Example: Pulmonology.

Section 2: Common Suffixes for Body Systems

-ology: Denoting the study or science of a particular body system or condition. Example: Dermatology (study of the skin).

-itis: Indicating inflammation of a particular body part or system. Example: Arthritis (inflammation of the joints).

-ectomy: Signifying the surgical removal of a body part or organ. Example: Appendectomy (surgical removal of the appendix).

-emia: Representing a condition of the blood. Example: Anemia (a condition characterized by a deficiency of red blood cells).

-pathy: Referring to a disease or abnormality in a particular body system. Example: Cardiomyopathy (disease of the heart muscle).

Section 3: Combined Prefixes and Suffixes for Body Systems

Neurology: Combines the prefix "neuro-" (nervous system) with the suffix "-ology" (the study of). It refers to the medical specialty that deals with the nervous system.

Hematology: Combines the prefix "hemo-" (blood) with the suffix "-ology" (the study of). It refers to the study of blood and blood-related disorders.

Gastroenteritis: Combines the prefix "gastro-" (stomach or gastrointestinal system) with the suffix "-itis" (inflammation). It denotes inflammation of the stomach and intestines.

Dermatopathology: Combines the root word "dermat" (skin) with the suffix "-pathy" (disease or abnormality) and the suffix "-ology" (the study of). It refers to the study of skin diseases and abnormalities.

Pulmonectomy: Combines the prefix "pulmo-" (lungs) with the suffix "-ectomy" (surgical removal). It denotes the surgical removal of a portion of the lung or a lung itself.

CHAPTER 9

Practice Exercises

To reinforce your understanding of medical terminology and its application in healthcare, this chapter offers a series of practice exercises. These exercises include identifying prefixes, suffixes, and root words, defining medical terms, and creating terms based on provided definitions. Engaging in these exercises will help you become more proficient in the language of healthcare.

Section 1: Identifying Prefixes, Suffixes, and Root Words

Exercise 1: Given the term "cardiomyopathy," identify the prefix, root word, and suffix in this medical term.

Exercise 2: In the term "gastrectomy," pinpoint the prefix, root word, and suffix.

Exercise 3: Analyze the term "neurology" to find the prefix, root word, and suffix.

Exercise 4: For the term "dermatologist," identify the prefix, root word, and suffix.

Section 2: Defining Medical Terms

Exercise 5: Define the term "hemorrhage."

Exercise 6: Provide a definition for "arthroscopy."

Exercise 7: Explain the meaning of "oncology."

Exercise 8: Define the term "pulmonary."

Section 3: Creating Medical Terms

Exercise 9: Using the root word "dermato-" (related to skin) and the suffix "-itis" (inflammation), create a medical term and provide its definition.

Exercise 10: Combine the prefix "gastro-" (related to the stomach) with the root word "entero-" (related to the intestines) and the suffix "-logy" (the study of) to form a medical term and define it.

Exercise 11: Form a medical term by combining the root word "cardio-" (related to the heart) with the suffix "-gram" (a record or image), and provide the definition of the term.

Exercise 12: Create a medical term by combining the prefix "neuro-" (related to the nervous system) with the root word "patho-" (related to disease) and the suffix "-logist" (a specialist in a field). Define the term you create.

CHAPTER 10

Medical Terminology in Practice

Medical terminology is not only a language for healthcare professionals but a vital tool for effective patient care, documentation, and communication. This chapter focuses on the practical application of medical terminology in various healthcare contexts, emphasizing its importance in daily medical practice.

Section 1: Medical Records and Documentation

Electronic Health Records (EHRs): How medical terminology is used in EHRs for accurate patient documentation and record-keeping.

Patient History and Charting: The role of medical terminology in documenting a patient's medical history, current condition, and treatment plan.

Section 2: Patient Consultations and Communication

Patient Education: The use of medical terminology to educate patients about their conditions, treatments, and medications.

Informed Consent: Explaining medical procedures and obtaining informed consent using clear and precise language.

Section 3: Diagnoses and Treatment

Diagnostic Terminology: The application of medical terminology in diagnosing conditions, interpreting test results, and discussing treatment options with patients.

Prescription and Medication Management: The use of medical

terms in prescribing medications, including dosages, routes, and frequency.

Section 4: Specialized Fields and Medical Teams

Interdisciplinary Collaboration: How healthcare professionals from different specialties communicate using medical terminology to provide comprehensive patient care.

Referrals and Consultations: Using precise terminology when referring patients to specialists for further evaluation and treatment.

Section 5: Emergency Medicine and Critical Care

Rapid Decision-Making: The critical role of medical terminology in urgent care settings, where quick and accurate communication is essential.

Emergency Medical Services (EMS): How EMS personnel use

medical terminology during emergencies to relay crucial information to healthcare providers.

Section 6: Medical Terminology in Telemedicine

Telehealth and Remote Consultations: The adaptation of medical terminology for telemedicine, where healthcare providers communicate with patients remotely.

Interoperability and Health Information Exchange: How standardized medical terminology facilitates data exchange between healthcare systems in telemedicine.

CHAPTER 11

Ethical and Cultural Considerations in Healthcare

Healthcare is not just a science; it's also a practice that involves ethics, cultural sensitivity, and respect for individual beliefs and values. This chapter explores the ethical and cultural aspects of healthcare and the importance of understanding and integrating these considerations into the practice of medicine.

Section 1: Medical Ethics

Patient Autonomy: The principle that patients have the right to make decisions about their own healthcare, including the use of medical terminology to explain choices and treatments.

Informed Consent: The ethical obligation to provide patients with clear and understandable information about their conditions, treatments, and procedures, using appropriate medical terminology.

Section 2: Cultural Competence

Cultural Awareness: The recognition of cultural diversity and the importance of understanding the cultural backgrounds and beliefs of patients.

Language Barriers: The challenges of communication when patients and healthcare providers speak different languages, and the use of medical terminology to bridge these gaps.

Section 3: Ethical Dilemmas

End-of-Life Care: The ethical considerations and communication strategies when discussing end-of-life decisions with patients and their families.

Confidentiality and Privacy: The ethical duty to maintain patient confidentiality and how to discuss sensitive issues using medical terminology.

Section 4: Special Populations and Cultural Sensitivity

Pediatric Patients: The importance of using age-appropriate medical terminology when communicating with children and their parents.

Geriatric Patients: Understanding the unique healthcare needs and challenges faced by elderly patients, and the use of medical terminology in their care.

Section 5: Diversity and Equity in Healthcare

Health Disparities: The impact of social, economic, and cultural factors on healthcare access and outcomes, and the role of healthcare providers in addressing these disparities.

Cultural Competence Training: The importance of ongoing education and training in cultural competence for healthcare professionals.

CHAPTER 12

Future Trends in Medical Terminology

The field of healthcare is continually evolving, and medical terminology is no exception. This chapter delves into the future trends and developments in medical terminology, including the influence of technology, emerging healthcare practices, and the importance of staying up-to-date in this dynamic field.

Section 1: Technology-Driven Advancements

Artificial Intelligence (AI): How AI is transforming medical terminology by improving medical coding, speech recognition, and natural language processing for EHRs.

Health Information Exchange (HIE): The role of standardized medical terminology in enhancing data interoperability and information exchange across healthcare systems.

Section 2: Precision Medicine and Genomics

Genomic Terminology: The impact of genomics on medical terminology, including the development of new terms for personalized medicine.

Pharmacogenomics: How genetics and medical terminology intersect to tailor drug treatments to individual genetic profiles.

Section 3: Telemedicine and Remote Healthcare

Telehealth Terminology: The expansion of medical terminology to include telehealth-specific terms, facilitating remote consultations and patient care.

Remote Monitoring and Wearables: The integration of medical terminology for wearable health devices and remote patient monitoring.

Section 4: Emerging Healthcare Practices

Regenerative Medicine: The development of new terminology to describe regenerative therapies, stem cell treatments, and tissue engineering.

Telepathology and Telediagnosis: The use of medical terminology in emerging practices that involve remote diagnosis and consultation for pathology.

Section 5: Patient-Centered Care and Health Literacy

Patient-Friendly Terminology: The trend toward simplifying medical terminology to enhance patient understanding and health literacy.

Shared Decision-Making: The role of medical terminology in shared decision-making between patients and healthcare providers.

Section 6: Globalization and Cross-Cultural Communication

International Classification of Diseases (ICD) Updates: How ICD coding systems adapt to global healthcare trends and emerging diseases.

Multilingual Healthcare: The importance of multilingual and culturally sensitive medical terminology to meet the needs of diverse patient populations.

ABOUT THE AUTHOR

Alex Usifo

Dr. Alex Usifo is a highly respected researcher with over two decades of experience in the field of medicine. I have made significant contributions to the medical field through her clinical work, research, and her role in mentoring the next generation of medical professionals. I have published numerous articles in reputable medical journals and has been at the forefront of groundbreaking research in areas such as cardiovascular medicine and preventive healthcare.

My motivation as an author of medical books is to bridge the gap between medical knowledge and patient understanding. She is deeply committed to making complex medical concepts accessible to the general public and to healthcare professionals seeking to expand their knowledge.

This book covers a wide range of medical topics, from comprehensive guides on specific medical conditions and their treatments to books focusing on wellness, nutrition, and lifestyle choices for maintaining optimal health. My works provide valuable insights for patients, caregivers, and healthcare practitioners alike.

As a medical author, my work serves as a valuable resource for those seeking to better understand medical conditions, treatment options, and the importance of maintaining good health. Her dedication to improving healthcare literacy and her contributions to medical literature have positively impacted countless lives.